Diabetic Daily Journal Log Book

Jenny Brown

Copyright © 2013 Jenny Brown

ISBN-13: 978-1492377573

DEDICATION

This e-book is dedicated to all the moms who work 24/7 to take care of their families with love and devotion. And also to our mothers, who taught us how to cook, take care of the house and our children.

If you leave a comment at
http://onlinebooks4you.blogspot.com/
The next time one of my Diabetic EBooks are FREE I will email you the information.

CONTENTS

If this book is found please return to:

My Name: _____

Phone: _____

Cell: _____

Address: _____

State: _____

Country: _____

MONTH ONE

The importance of recording your blood glucose is so very important and I am certain your doctor has stressed this to you repeatedly.

Therefore Log books and data collection are a crucial part of keeping your diabetes under control. When you write down the numbers it is easier to see your blood sugar patterns. and know when you are on target.

Perhaps more important is to know when your glucose is going the wrong direction. Most people trying to remember multiple blood sugar numbers, and what was happening at the same time as the blood sugar check is difficult, and often leads to false assumptions and bad decisions.

Everyone is different and depending on your type of physician prescribed treatment you may need to check your blood sugar once every few days or even multiple times a day.

If you are treated with a strict diet, and your blood sugar is under control, you may only need to check your blood glucose every few days. However, if your blood sugar is not well controlled and or you are starting medications or taking insulin or pills that increase your insulin levels you should check multiple times a day.

Remember when taking insulin, you also need to record your insulin dose, and usually your food and carbohydrate intake and activity level.

The simple method of tracking your blood sugar at various times on different days is suitable when your treatment doesn't change or you are not at risk of having a low blood sugar.

When you want to understand how your blood sugar is responding to different foods, activities and medication you will need many more reading and keeping track of what you're eating, sugar, the carb and fat levels. From your record keeping many important things can be revealed to you and most importantly your doctor.

A good and complex log book records the most important variables that affect the blood sugar, including:

a. blood sugar level

b. type and dose of medications or insulin

c. time of day

d. amount of carbohydrate or sugar eaten

e. food diary (and be honest)

f. type and duration of exercise

g. unusual events such as medications or stresses

So much can be benefited by recording this data and I encourage you to give it a try for 90 days and you will be amazed at the benefits you achieve. I was in awe at the pattern that developed from consistent 30 minutes on the treadmill. My glucose came down undeniably.

NOTES
This is where you tell about the foods that you ate and were not good choices. Tell about your exercise or lack there off. Include details that will reveal the problem areas.

Date: Day:	AM	AM	AM	AM	AM	AM	PM	PM	PM	PM	PM	PM	PM	PM	PM	PM
Glucose																
A1C1																
Carb Grams																
Fat Grams																
Basal Rate																
Ketones																

NOTES
This is where you tell about the foods that you ate and were not good choices. Tell about your exercise or lack there off. Include details that will reveal the problem areas.

Date: Day:	AM	AM	AM	AM	AM	AM	PM	PM	PM	PM	PM	PM	PM	PM	PM	PM
Glucose																
A1C1																
Carb Grams																
Fat Grams																
Basal Rate																
Ketones																

NOTES
This is where you tell about the foods that you ate and were not good choices. Tell about your exercise or lack there off. Include details that will reveal the problem areas.

Date: Day:	AM	AM	AM	AM	AM	AM	PM	PM	PM	PM	PM	PM	PM	PM	PM	PM
Glucose																
A1C1																
Carb Grams																
Fat Grams																
Basal Rate																
Ketones																

NOTES

This is where you tell about the foods that you ate and were not good choices. Tell about your exercise or lack there off. Include details that will reveal the problem areas.

Date: Day:	AM	AM	AM	AM	AM	AM	PM	PM	PM	PM	PM	PM	PM	PM	PM	PM
Glucose																
A1C1																
Carb Grams																
Fat Grams																
Basal Rate																
Ketones																

NOTES
This is where you tell about the foods that you ate and were not good choices. Tell about your exercise or lack there off. Include details that will reveal the problem areas.

Date: Day:	AM	AM	AM	AM	AM	AM	PM	PM	PM	PM	PM	PM	PM	PM	PM	PM
Glucose																
A1C1																
Carb Grams																
Fat Grams																
Basal Rate																
Ketones																

NOTES
This is whcrc you tell about the foods that you ate and were not good choices. Tell about your exercise or lack there off. Include details that will reveal the problem areas.

Date: Day:	AM	AM	AM	AM	AM	AM	PM	PM	PM	PM	PM	PM	PM	PM	PM	PM
Glucose																
A1C1																
Carb Grams																
Fat Grams																
Basal Rate																
Ketones																

NOTES
This is where you tell about the foods that you ate and were not good choices. Tell about your exercise or lack there off. Include details that will reveal the problem areas.

Date: Day:	AM	AM	AM	AM	AM	AM	PM	PM	PM	PM	PM	PM	PM	PM	PM	PM
Glucose																
A1C1																
Carb Grams																
Fat Grams																
Basal Rate																
Ketones																

NOTES

This is where you tell about the foods that you ate and were not good choices. Tell about your exercise or lack there off. Include details that will reveal the problem areas.

Date: Day:	A M	A M	A M	A M	A M	A M	P M	P M	P M	P M	P M	P M	P M	P M	P M	P M
Glucose																
A1C1																
Carb Grams																
Fat Grams																
Basal Rate																
Ketones																

NOTES

This is where you tell about the foods that you ate and were not good choices. Tell about your exercise or lack there off. Include details that will reveal the problem areas.

Date: Day:	A M	A M	A M	A M	A M	A M	P M	P M	P M	P M	P M	P M	P M	P M	P M	P M
Glucose																
A1C1																
Carb Grams																
Fat Grams																
Basal Rate																
Ketones																

NOTES
This is where you tell about the foods that you ate and were not good choices. Tell about your exercise or lack there off. Include details that will reveal the problem areas.

Date: Day:	A M	A M	A M	A M	A M	A M	P M	P M	P M	P M	P M	P M	P M	P M	P M	P M
Glucose																
A1C1																
Carb Grams																
Fat Grams																
Basal Rate																
Ketones																

NOTES

This is where you tell about the foods that you ate and were not good choices. Tell about your exercise or lack there off. Include details that will reveal the problem areas.

Date: Day:	A M	A M	A M	A M	A M	A M	P M	P M	P M	P M	P M	P M	P M	P M	P M	P M
Glucose																
A1C1																
Carb Grams																
Fat Grams																
Basal Rate																
Ketones																

NOTES

This is where you tell about the foods that you ate and were not good choices. Tell about your exercise or lack there off. Include details that will reveal the problem areas.

Date: Day:	A M	A M	A M	A M	A M	A M	P M	P M	P M	P M	P M	P M	P M	P M	P M	P M
Glucose																
A1C1																
Carb Grams																
Fat Grams																
Basal Rate																
Ketones																

NOTES

This is where you tell about the foods that you ate and were not good choices. Tell about your exercise or lack there off. Include details that will reveal the problem areas.

Date: Day:	A M	A M	A M	A M	A M	A M	P M	P M	P M	P M	P M	P M	P M	P M	P M	P M
Glucose																
A1C1																
Carb Grams																
Fat Grams																
Basal Rate																
Ketones																

NOTES
This is where you tell about the foods that you ate and were not good choices. Tell about your exercise or lack there off. Include details that will reveal the problem areas.

Date: Day:	A M	A M	A M	A M	A M	A M	P M	P M	P M	P M	P M	P M	P M	P M	P M	P M
Glucose																
A1C1																
Carb Grams																
Fat Grams																
Basal Rate																
Ketones																

NOTES

This is where you tell about the foods that you ate and were not good choices. Tell about your exercise or lack there off. Include details that will reveal the problem areas.

Date: Day:	A M	A M	A M	A M	A M	A M	P M	P M	P M	P M	P M	P M	P M	P M	P M	P M
Glucose																
A1C1																
Carb Grams																
Fat Grams																
Basal Rate																
Ketones																

NOTES
This is where you tell about the foods that you ate and were not good choices. Tell about your exercise or lack there off. Include details that will reveal the problem areas.

Date: Day:	A M	A M	A M	A M	A M	A M	P M	P M	P M	P M	P M	P M	P M	P M	P M	P M
Glucose																
A1C1																
Carb Grams																
Fat Grams																
Basal Rate																
Ketones																

NOTES
This is where you tell about the foods that you ate and were not good choices. Tell about your exercise or lack there off. Include details that will reveal the problem areas.

Date: Day:	A M	A M	A M	A M	A M	A M	P M	P M	P M	P M	P M	P M	P M	P M	P M	P M
Glucose																
A1C1																
Carb Grams																
Fat Grams																
Basal Rate																
Ketones																

NOTES
This is where you tell about the foods that you ate and were not good choices. Tell about your exercise or lack there off. Include details that will reveal the problem areas.

Date: Day:	A M	A M	A M	A M	A M	A M	P M	P M	P M	P M	P M	P M	P M	P M	P M	P M
Glucose																
A1C1																
Carb Grams																
Fat Grams																
Basal Rate																
Ketones																

NOTES
This is where you tell about the foods that you ate and were not good choices. Tell about your exercise or lack there off. Include details that will reveal the problem areas.

Date: Day:	A M	A M	A M	A M	A M	A M	P M	P M	P M	P M	P M	P M	P M	P M	P M	P M
Glucose																
A1C1																
Carb Grams																
Fat Grams																
Basal Rate																
Ketones																

NOTES

This is where you tell about the foods that you ate and were not good choices. Tell about your exercise or lack there off. Include details that will reveal the problem areas.

Date: Day:	A M	A M	A M	A M	A M	A M	P M	P M	P M	P M	P M	P M	P M	P M	P M	P M
Glucose																
A1C1																
Carb Grams																
Fat Grams																
Basal Rate																
Ketones																

NOTES

This is where you tell about the foods that you ate and were not good choices. Tell about your exercise or lack there off. Include details that will reveal the problem areas.

Date: Day:	A M	A M	A M	A M	A M	A M	P M	P M	P M	P M	P M	P M	P M	P M	P M	P M
Glucose																
A1C1																
Carb Grams																
Fat Grams																
Basal Rate																
Ketones																

NOTES

This is where you tell about the foods that you ate and were not good choices. Tell about your exercise or lack there off. Include details that will reveal the problem areas.

Date: Day:	A M	A M	A M	A M	A M	A M	P M	P M	P M	P M	P M	P M	P M	P M	P M	P M
Glucose																
A1C1																
Carb Grams																
Fat Grams																
Basal Rate																
Ketones																

NOTES
This is where you tell about the foods that you ate and were not good choices. Tell about your exercise or lack there off. Include details that will reveal the problem areas.

Date: Day:	A M	A M	A M	A M	A M	A M	P M	P M	P M	P M	P M	P M	P M	P M	P M	P M
Glucose																
A1C1																
Carb Grams																
Fat Grams																
Basal Rate																
Ketones																

NOTES

This is where you tell about the foods that you ate and were not good choices. Tell about your exercise or lack there off. Include details that will reveal the problem areas.

Date: Day:	A M	A M	A M	A M	A M	A M	P M	P M	P M	P M	P M	P M	P M	P M	P M	P M
Glucose																
A1C1																
Carb Grams																
Fat Grams																
Basal Rate																
Ketones																

NOTES
This is where you tell about the foods that you ate and were not good choices. Tell about your exercise or lack there off. Include details that will reveal the problem areas.

Date: Day:	A M	A M	A M	A M	A M	A M	P M	P M	P M	P M	P M	P M	P M	P M	P M	P M
Glucose																
A1C1																
Carb Grams																
Fat Grams																
Basal Rate																
Ketones																

NOTES
This is where you tell about the foods that you ate and were not good choices. Tell about your exercise or lack there off. Include details that will reveal the problem areas.

Date: Day:	A M	A M	A M	A M	A M	A M	P M	P M	P M	P M	P M	P M	P M	P M	P M	P M
Glucose																
A1C1																
Carb Grams																
Fat Grams																
Basal Rate																
Ketones																

NOTES

This is where you tell about the foods that you ate and were not good choices. Tell about your exercise or lack there off. Include details that will reveal the problem areas.

Date: Day:	A M	A M	A M	A M	A M	A M	P M	P M	P M	P M	P M	P M	P M	P M	P M	P M
Glucose																
A1C1																
Carb Grams																
Fat Grams																
Basal Rate																
Ketones																

NOTES

This is where you tell about the foods that you ate and were not good choices. Tell about your exercise or lack there off. Include details that will reveal the problem areas.

Date: Day:	A M	A M	A M	A M	A M	A M	P M	P M	P M	P M	P M	P M	P M	P M	P M	P M
Glucose																
A1C1																
Carb Grams																
Fat Grams																
Basal Rate																
Ketones																

NOTES
This is where you tell about the foods that you ate and were not good choices. Tell about your exercise or lack there off. Include details that will reveal the problem areas.

Date: Day:	A M	A M	A M	A M	A M	A M	P M	P M	P M	P M	P M	P M	P M	P M	P M	P M
Glucose																
A1C1																
Carb Grams																
Fat Grams																
Basal Rate																
Ketones																

NOTES
This is where you tell about the foods that you ate and were not good choices. Tell about your exercise or lack there off. Include details that will reveal the problem areas.

Date: Day:	A M	A M	A M	A M	A M	A M	P M	P M	P M	P M	P M	P M	P M	P M	P M	P M
Glucose																
A1C1																
Carb Grams																
Fat Grams																
Basal Rate																
Ketones																

NOTES
This is where you tell about the foods that you ate and were not good choices. Tell about your exercise or lack there off. Include details that will reveal the problem areas.

Date: Day:	A M	A M	A M	A M	A M	A M	P M	P M	P M	P M	P M	P M	P M	P M	P M	P M
Glucose																
A1C1																
Carb Grams																
Fat Grams																
Basal Rate																
Ketones																

MONTH TWO

Congratulations you have completed your first month. How did you do with your data? Keep up the great work and be consistent and there will be results in improved glucose and better health.

NOTES

This is where you tell about the foods that you ate and were not good choices. Tell about your exercise or lack there off. Include details that will reveal the problem areas.

Date:																
Day:	A M	A M	A M	A M	A M	A M	P M	P M	P M	P M	P M	P M	P M	P M	P M	P M
Glucose																
A1C1																
Carb Grams																
Fat Grams																
Basal Rate																
Ketones																

NOTES

This is where you tell about the foods that you ate and were not good choices. Tell about your exercise or lack there off. Include details that will reveal the problem areas.

Date: Day:	A M	A M	A M	A M	A M	A M	P M	P M	P M	P M	P M	P M	P M	P M	P M	P M
Glucose																
A1C1																
Carb Grams																
Fat Grams																
Basal Rate																
Ketones																

NOTES

This is where you tell about the foods that you ate and were not good choices. Tell about your exercise or lack there off. Include details that will reveal the problem areas.

Date: Day:	A M	A M	A M	A M	A M	A M	P M	P M	P M	P M	P M	P M	P M	P M	P M	P M
Glucose																
A1C1																
Carb Grams																
Fat Grams																
Basal Rate																
Ketones																

NOTES

This is where you tell about the foods that you ate and were not good choices. Tell about your exercise or lack there off. Include details that will reveal the problem areas.

Date: Day:	A M	A M	A M	A M	A M	A M	P M	P M	P M	P M	P M	P M	P M	P M	P M	P M
Glucose																
A1C1																
Carb Grams																
Fat Grams																
Basal Rate																
Ketones																

NOTES

This is where you tell about the foods that you ate and were not good choices. Tell about your exercise or lack there off. Include details that will reveal the problem areas.

Date: Day:	A M	A M	A M	A M	A M	A M	P M	P M	P M	P M	P M	P M	P M	P M	P M	P M
Glucose																
A1C1																
Carb Grams																
Fat Grams																
Basal Rate																
Ketones																

NOTES

This is where you tell about the foods that you ate and were not good choices. Tell about your exercise or lack there off. Include details that will reveal the problem areas.

Date: Day:	A M	A M	A M	A M	A M	A M	P M	P M	P M	P M	P M	P M	P M	P M	P M	P M
Glucose																
A1C1																
Carb Grams																
Fat Grams																
Basal Rate																
Ketones																

NOTES
This is where you tell about the foods that you ate and were not good choices. Tell about your exercise or lack there off. Include details that will reveal the problem areas.

Date: Day:	A M	A M	A M	A M	A M	A M	P M	P M	P M	P M	P M	P M	P M	P M	P M	P M
Glucose																
A1C1																
Carb Grams																
Fat Grams																
Basal Rate																
Ketones																

NOTES

This is where you tell about the foods that you ate and were not good choices. Tell about your exercise or lack there off. Include details that will reveal the problem areas.

Date: Day:	A M	A M	A M	A M	A M	A M	P M	P M	P M	P M	P M	P M	P M	P M	P M	P M
Glucose																
A1C1																
Carb Grams																
Fat Grams																
Basal Rate																
Ketones																

NOTES
This is where you tell about the foods that you ate and were not good choices. Tell about your exercise or lack there off. Include details that will reveal the problem areas.

Date: Day:	A M	A M	A M	A M	A M	A M	P M	P M	P M	P M	P M	P M	P M	P M	P M	P M
Glucose																
A1C1																
Carb Grams																
Fat Grams																
Basal Rate																
Ketones																

NOTES

This is where you tell about the foods that you ate and were not good choices. Tell about your exercise or lack there off. Include details that will reveal the problem areas.

Date: Day:	A M	A M	A M	A M	A M	A M	P M	P M	P M	P M	P M	P M	P M	P M	P M	P M
Glucose																
A1C1																
Carb Grams																
Fat Grams																
Basal Rate																
Ketones																

NOTES

This is where you tell about the foods that you ate and were not good choices. Tell about your exercise or lack there off. Include details that will reveal the problem areas.

Date: Day:	A M	A M	A M	A M	A M	A M	P M	P M	P M	P M	P M	P M	P M	P M	P M	P M
Glucose																
A1C1																
Carb Grams																
Fat Grams																
Basal Rate																
Ketones																

NOTES

This is where you tell about the foods that you ate and were not good choices. Tell about your exercise or lack there off. Include details that will reveal the problem areas.

Date: Day:	A M	A M	A M	A M	A M	A M	P M	P M	P M	P M	P M	P M	P M	P M	P M	P M
Glucose																
A1C1																
Carb Grams																
Fat Grams																
Basal Rate																
Ketones																

NOTES

This is where you tell about the foods that you ate and were not good choices. Tell about your exercise or lack there off. Include details that will reveal the problem areas.

Date: Day:	A M	A M	A M	A M	A M	A M	P M	P M	P M	P M	P M	P M	P M	P M	P M	P M
Glucose																
A1C1																
Carb Grams																
Fat Grams																
Basal Rate																
Ketones																

NOTES
This is where you tell about the foods that you ate and were not good choices. Tell about your exercise or lack there off. Include details that will reveal the problem areas.

Date: Day:	A M	A M	A M	A M	A M	A M	P M	P M	P M	P M	P M	P M	P M	P M	P M	P M
Glucose																
A1C1																
Carb Grams																
Fat Grams																
Basal Rate																
Ketones																

NOTES

This is where you tell about the foods that you ate and were not good choices. Tell about your exercise or lack there off. Include details that will reveal the problem areas.

Date: Day:	A M	A M	A M	A M	A M	A M	P M	P M	P M	P M	P M	P M	P M	P M	P M	P M
Glucose																
A1C1																
Carb Grams																
Fat Grams																
Basal Rate																
Ketones																

NOTES

This is where you tell about the foods that you ate and were not good choices. Tell about your exercise or lack there off. Include details that will reveal the problem areas.

Date: / Day:	A M	A M	A M	A M	A M	A M	P M	P M	P M	P M	P M	P M	P M	P M	P M	P M
Glucose																
A1C1																
Carb Grams																
Fat Grams																
Basal Rate																
Ketones																

NOTES

This is where you tell about the foods that you ate and were not good choices. Tell about your exercise or lack there off. Include details that will reveal the problem areas.

Date: Day:	A M	A M	A M	A M	A M	A M	P M	P M	P M	P M	P M	P M	P M	P M	P M	P M
Glucose																
A1C1																
Carb Grams																
Fat Grams																
Basal Rate																
Ketones																

NOTES

This is where you tell about the foods that you ate and were not good choices. Tell about your exercise or lack there off. Include details that will reveal the problem areas.

Date: Day:	A M	A M	A M	A M	A M	A M	P M	P M	P M	P M	P M	P M	P M	P M	P M	P M
Glucose																
A1C1																
Carb Grams																
Fat Grams																
Basal Rate																
Ketones																

NOTES
This is where you tell about the foods that you ate and were not good choices. Tell about your exercise or lack there off. Include details that will reveal the problem areas.

Date: Day:	A M	A M	A M	A M	A M	A M	P M	P M	P M	P M	P M	P M	P M	P M	P M	P M
Glucose																
A1C1																
Carb Grams																
Fat Grams																
Basal Rate																
Ketones																

NOTES

This is where you tell about the foods that you ate and were not good choices. Tell about your exercise or lack there off. Include details that will reveal the problem areas.

Date: Day:	A M	A M	A M	A M	A M	A M	P M	P M	P M	P M	P M	P M	P M	P M	P M	P M
Glucose																
A1C1																
Carb Grams																
Fat Grams																
Basal Rate																
Ketones																

NOTES
This is where you tell about the foods that you ate and were not good choices. Tell about your exercise or lack there off. Include details that will reveal the problem areas.

Date: Day:	A M	A M	A M	A M	A M	A M	P M	P M	P M	P M	P M	P M	P M	P M	P M	P M
Glucose																
A1C1																
Carb Grams																
Fat Grams																
Basal Rate																
Ketones																

NOTES

This is where you tell about the foods that you ate and were not good choices. Tell about your exercise or lack there off. Include details that will reveal the problem areas.

Date: Day:	A M	A M	A M	A M	A M	A M	P M	P M	P M	P M	P M	P M	P M	P M	P M	P M
Glucose																
A1C1																
Carb Grams																
Fat Grams																
Basal Rate																
Ketones																

NOTES

This is where you tell about the foods that you ate and were not good choices. Tell about your exercise or lack there off. Include details that will reveal the problem areas.

Date: Day:	A M	A M	A M	A M	A M	A M	P M	P M	P M	P M	P M	P M	P M	P M	P M	P M
Glucose																
A1C1																
Carb Grams																
Fat Grams																
Basal Rate																
Ketones																

NOTES
This is where you tell about the foods that you ate and
were not good choices. Tell about your exercise or lack
there off. Include details that will reveal the problem areas.

Date: Day:	A M	A M	A M	A M	A M	A M	P M	P M	P M	P M	P M	P M	P M	P M	P M	P M
Glucose																
A1C1																
Carb Grams																
Fat Grams																
Basal Rate																
Ketones																

NOTES
This is where you tell about the foods that you ate and were not good choices. Tell about your exercise or lack there off. Include details that will reveal the problem areas.

Date: Day:	A M	A M	A M	A M	A M	A M	P M	P M	P M	P M	P M	P M	P M	P M	P M	P M
Glucose																
A1C1																
Carb Grams																
Fat Grams																
Basal Rate																
Ketones																

NOTES

This is where you tell about the foods that you ate and were not good choices. Tell about your exercise or lack there off. Include details that will reveal the problem areas.

Date: Day:	A M	A M	A M	A M	A M	A M	P M	P M	P M	P M	P M	P M	P M	P M	P M	P M
Glucose																
A1C1																
Carb Grams																
Fat Grams																
Basal Rate																
Ketones																

NOTES
This is where you tell about the foods that you ate and were not good choices. Tell about your exercise or lack there off. Include details that will reveal the problem areas.

Date: Day:	A M	A M	A M	A M	A M	A M	P M	P M	P M	P M	P M	P M	P M	P M	P M	P M
Glucose																
A1C1																
Carb Grams																
Fat Grams																
Basal Rate																
Ketones																

NOTES

This is where you tell about the foods that you ate and were not good choices. Tell about your exercise or lack there off. Include details that will reveal the problem areas.

Date: Day:	A M	A M	A M	A M	A M	A M	P M	P M	P M	P M	P M	P M	P M	P M	P M	P M
Glucose																
A1C1																
Carb Grams																
Fat Grams																
Basal Rate																
Ketones																

NOTES

This is where you tell about the foods that you ate and were not good choices. Tell about your exercise or lack there off. Include details that will reveal the problem areas.

Date: Day:	A M	A M	A M	A M	A M	A M	P M	P M	P M	P M	P M	P M	P M	P M	P M	P M
Glucose																
A1C1																
Carb Grams																
Fat Grams																
Basal Rate																
Ketones																

NOTES
This is where you tell about the foods that you ate and were not good choices. Tell about your exercise or lack there off. Include details that will reveal the problem areas.

Date: Day:	AM	AM	AM	AM	AM	AM	PM	PM	PM	PM	PM	PM	PM	PM	PM	PM
Glucose																
A1C1																
Carb Grams																
Fat Grams																
Basal Rate																
Ketones																

NOTES
This is where you tell about the foods that you ate and were not good choices. Tell about your exercise or lack there off. Include details that will reveal the problem areas.

Date: Day:	AM	AM	AM	AM	AM	AM	PM	PM	PM	PM	PM	PM	PM	PM	PM	PM
Glucose																
A1C1																
Carb Grams																
Fat Grams																
Basal Rate																
Ketones																

MONTH THREE

Congratulations you have completed your first month. How did you do with your data? Keep up the great work and be consistent and there will be results in improved glucose and better health.

NOTES

This is where you tell about the foods that you ate and were not good choices. Tell about your exercise or lack there off. Include details that will reveal the problem areas.

Date: Day:	A M	A M	A M	A M	A M	A M	P M	P M	P M	P M	P M	P M	P M	P M	P M	P M
Glucose																
A1C1																
Carb Grams																
Fat Grams																
Basal Rate																
Ketones																

NOTES

This is where you tell about the foods that you ate and were not good choices. Tell about your exercise or lack there off. Include details that will reveal the problem areas.

Date: Day:	AM	AM	AM	AM	AM	AM	PM	PM	PM	PM	PM	PM	PM	PM	PM	PM
Glucose																
A1C1																
Carb Grams																
Fat Grams																
Basal Rate																
Ketones																

NOTES
This is where you tell about the foods that you ate and were not good choices. Tell about your exercise or lack there off. Include details that will reveal the problem areas.

Date: Day:	AM	AM	AM	AM	AM	AM	PM	PM	PM	PM	PM	PM	PM	PM	PM	PM
Glucose																
A1C1																
Carb Grams																
Fat Grams																
Basal Rate																
Ketones																

NOTES

This is where you tell about the foods that you ate and were not good choices. Tell about your exercise or lack there off. Include details that will reveal the problem areas.

Date: Day:	A M	A M	A M	A M	A M	A M	P M	P M	P M	P M	P M	P M	P M	P M	P M	P M
Glucose																
A1C1																
Carb Grams																
Fat Grams																
Basal Rate																
Ketones																

NOTES
This is where you tell about the foods that you ate and were not good choices. Tell about your exercise or lack there off. Include details that will reveal the problem areas.

Date: Day:	A M	A M	A M	A M	A M	A M	P M	P M	P M	P M	P M	P M	P M	P M	P M	P M
Glucose																
A1C1																
Carb Grams																
Fat Grams																
Basal Rate																
Ketones																

NOTES

This is where you tell about the foods that you ate and were not good choices. Tell about your exercise or lack there off. Include details that will reveal the problem areas.

Date: Day:	A M	A M	A M	A M	A M	A M	P M	P M	P M	P M	P M	P M	P M	P M	P M	P M
Glucose																
A1C1																
Carb Grams																
Fat Grams																
Basal Rate																
Ketones																

NOTES

This is where you tell about the foods that you ate and were not good choices. Tell about your exercise or lack there off. Include details that will reveal the problem areas.

Date: Day:	A M	A M	A M	A M	A M	A M	P M	P M	P M	P M	P M	P M	P M	P M	P M	P M
Glucose																
A1C1																
Carb Grams																
Fat Grams																
Basal Rate																
Ketones																

NOTES
This is where you tell about the foods that you ate and were not good choices. Tell about your exercise or lack there off. Include details that will reveal the problem areas.

Date: Day:	A M	A M	A M	A M	A M	A M	P M	P M	P M	P M	P M	P M	P M	P M	P M	P M
Glucose																
A1C1																
Carb Grams																
Fat Grams																
Basal Rate																
Ketones																

NOTES

This is where you tell about the foods that you ate and were not good choices. Tell about your exercise or lack there off. Include details that will reveal the problem areas.

Date: Day:	A M	A M	A M	A M	A M	A M	P M	P M	P M	P M	P M	P M	P M	P M	P M	P M
Glucose																
A1C1																
Carb Grams																
Fat Grams																
Basal Rate																
Ketones																

NOTES
This is where you tell about the foods that you ate and were not good choices. Tell about your exercise or lack there off. Include details that will reveal the problem areas.

Date: Day:	A M	A M	A M	A M	A M	A M	P M	P M	P M	P M	P M	P M	P M	P M	P M	P M
Glucose																
A1C1																
Carb Grams																
Fat Grams																
Basal Rate																
Ketones																

NOTES
This is where you tell about the foods that you ate and were not good choices. Tell about your exercise or lack there off. Include details that will reveal the problem areas.

Date: Day:	A M	A M	A M	A M	A M	A M	P M	P M	P M	P M	P M	P M	P M	P M	P M	P M
Glucose																
A1C1																
Carb Grams																
Fat Grams																
Basal Rate																
Ketones																

NOTES

This is where you tell about the foods that you atc and were not good choices. Tell about your exercise or lack there off. Include details that will reveal the problem areas.

Date: Day:	A M	A M	A M	A M	A M	A M	P M	P M	P M	P M	P M	P M	P M	P M	P M	P M
Glucose																
A1C1																
Carb Grams																
Fat Grams																
Basal Rate																
Ketones																

NOTES

This is where you tell about the foods that you ate and were not good choices. Tell about your exercise or lack there off. Include details that will reveal the problem areas.

Date: Day:	A M	A M	A M	A M	A M	A M	P M	P M	P M	P M	P M	P M	P M	P M	P M	P M
Glucose																
A1C1																
Carb Grams																
Fat Grams																
Basal Rate																
Ketones																

NOTES

This is where you tell about the foods that you ate and were not good choices. Tell about your exercise or lack there off. Include details that will reveal the problem areas.

Date: Day:	A M	A M	A M	A M	A M	A M	P M	P M	P M	P M	P M	P M	P M	P M	P M	P M
Glucose																
A1C1																
Carb Grams																
Fat Grams																
Basal Rate																
Ketones																

NOTES

This is where you tell about the foods that you ate and were not good choices. Tell about your exercise or lack there off. Include details that will reveal the problem areas.

Date: Day:	A M	A M	A M	A M	A M	A M	P M	P M	P M	P M	P M	P M	P M	P M	P M	P M
Glucose																
A1C1																
Carb Grams																
Fat Grams																
Basal Rate																
Ketones																

NOTES
This is where you tell about the foods that you ate and were not good choices. Tell about your exercise or lack there off. Include details that will reveal the problem areas.

Date: Day:	A M	A M	A M	A M	A M	A M	P M	P M	P M	P M	P M	P M	P M	P M	P M	P M
Glucose																
A1C1																
Carb Grams																
Fat Grams																
Basal Rate																
Ketones																

NOTES
This is where you tell about the foods that you ate and were not good choices. Tell about your exercise or lack there off. Include details that will reveal the problem areas.

Date: Day:	A M	A M	A M	A M	A M	A M	P M	P M	P M	P M	P M	P M	P M	P M	P M	P M
Glucose																
A1C1																
Carb Grams																
Fat Grams																
Basal Rate																
Ketones																

NOTES

This is where you tell about the foods that you ate and were not good choices. Tell about your exercise or lack there off. Include details that will reveal the problem areas.

Date: Day:	A M	A M	A M	A M	A M	A M	P M	P M	P M	P M	P M	P M	P M	P M	P M	P M
Glucose																
A1C1																
Carb Grams																
Fat Grams																
Basal Rate																
Ketones																

NOTES
This is where you tell about the foods that you ate and were not good choices. Tell about your exercise or lack there off. Include details that will reveal the problem areas.

Date: Day:	A M	A M	A M	A M	A M	A M	P M	P M	P M	P M	P M	P M	P M	P M	P M	P M
Glucose																
A1C1																
Carb Grams																
Fat Grams																
Basal Rate																
Ketones																

NOTES

This is where you tell about the foods that you ate and were not good choices. Tell about your exercise or lack there off. Include details that will reveal the problem areas.

Date: Day:	A M	A M	A M	A M	A M	A M	P M	P M	P M	P M	P M	P M	P M	P M	P M	P M
Glucose																
A1C1																
Carb Grams																
Fat Grams																
Basal Rate																
Ketones																

NOTES

This is where you tell about the foods that you ate and were not good choices. Tell about your exercise or lack there off. Include details that will reveal the problem areas.

Date: Day:	AM	AM	AM	AM	AM	AM	PM	PM	PM	PM	PM	PM	PM	PM	PM	PM
Glucose																
A1C1																
Carb Grams																
Fat Grams																
Basal Rate																
Ketones																

NOTES

This is where you tell about the foods that you ate and were not good choices. Tell about your exercise or lack there off. Include details that will reveal the problem areas.

Date: Day:	A M	A M	A M	A M	A M	A M	P M	P M	P M	P M	P M	P M	P M	P M	P M	P M
Glucose																
A1C1																
Carb Grams																
Fat Grams																
Basal Rate																
Ketones																

NOTES
This is where you tell about the foods that you ate and were not good choices. Tell about your exercise or lack there off. Include details that will reveal the problem areas.

Date: Day:	A M	A M	A M	A M	A M	A M	P M	P M	P M	P M	P M	P M	P M	P M	P M	P M
Glucose																
A1C1																
Carb Grams																
Fat Grams																
Basal Rate																
Ketones																

NOTES

This is where you tell about the foods that you ate and were not good choices. Tell about your exercise or lack there off. Include details that will reveal the problem areas.

Date: Day:	A M	A M	A M	A M	A M	A M	P M	P M	P M	P M	P M	P M	P M	P M	P M	P M
Glucose																
A1C1																
Carb Grams																
Fat Grams																
Basal Rate																
Ketones																

NOTES
This is where you tell about the foods that you ate and were not good choices. Tell about your exercise or lack there off. Include details that will reveal the problem areas.

Date: Day:	A M	A M	A M	A M	A M	A M	P M	P M	P M	P M	P M	P M	P M	P M	P M	P M
Glucose																
A1C1																
Carb Grams																
Fat Grams																
Basal Rate																
Ketones																

NOTES
This is where you tell about the foods that you ate and were not good choices. Tell about your exercise or lack there off. Include details that will reveal the problem areas.

Date: Day:	A M	A M	A M	A M	A M	A M	P M	P M	P M	P M	P M	P M	P M	P M	P M	P M
Glucose																
A1C1																
Carb Grams																
Fat Grams																
Basal Rate																
Ketones																

NOTES

This is where you tell about the foods that you ate and were not good choices. Tell about your exercise or lack there off. Include details that will reveal the problem areas.

Date: Day:	A M	A M	A M	A M	A M	A M	P M	P M	P M	P M	P M	P M	P M	P M	P M	P M
Glucose																
A1C1																
Carb Grams																
Fat Grams																
Basal Rate																
Ketones																

NOTES

This is where you tell about the foods that you ate and were not good choices. Tell about your exercise or lack there off. Include details that will reveal the problem areas.

Date: Day:	A M	A M	A M	A M	A M	A M	P M	P M	P M	P M	P M	P M	P M	P M	P M	P M
Glucose																
A1C1																
Carb Grams																
Fat Grams																
Basal Rate																
Ketones																

NOTES

This is where you tell about the foods that you ate and were not good choices. Tell about your exercise or lack there off. Include details that will reveal the problem areas.

Date: Day:	A M	A M	A M	A M	A M	A M	P M	P M	P M	P M	P M	P M	P M	P M	P M	P M
Glucose																
A1C1																
Carb Grams																
Fat Grams																
Basal Rate																
Ketones																

NOTES

This is where you tell about the foods that you ate and were not good choices. Tell about your exercise or lack there off. Include details that will reveal the problem areas.

Date: Day:	A M	A M	A M	A M	A M	A M	P M	P M	P M	P M	P M	P M	P M	P M	P M	P M
Glucose																
A1C1																
Carb Grams																
Fat Grams																
Basal Rate																
Ketones																

NOTES

This is where you tell about the foods that you ate and were not good choices. Tell about your exercise or lack there off. Include details that will reveal the problem areas.

Date: Day:	A M	A M	A M	A M	A M	A M	P M	P M	P M	P M	P M	P M	P M	P M	P M	P M
Glucose																
A1C1																
Carb Grams																
Fat Grams																
Basal Rate																
Ketones																

MONTH FOUR

Congratulations you are starting month number three and great things are ahead for your health!

NOTES

This is where you tell about the foods that you ate and were not good choices. Tell about your exercise or lack there off. Include details that will reveal the problem areas.

Date: Day:	A M	A M	A M	A M	A M	A M	P M	P M	P M	P M	P M	P M	P M	P M	P M	P M
Glucose																
A1C1																
Carb Grams																
Fat Grams																
Basal Rate																
Ketones																

NOTES

This is where you tell about the foods that you ate and were not good choices. Tell about your exercise or lack there off. Include details that will reveal the problem areas.

Date: Day:	A M	A M	A M	A M	A M	A M	P M	P M	P M	P M	P M	P M	P M	P M	P M	P M
Glucose																
A1C1																
Carb Grams																
Fat Grams																
Basal Rate																
Ketones																

NOTES
This is where you tell about the foods that you ate and were not good choices. Tell about your exercise or lack there off. Include details that will reveal the problem areas.

Date: Day:	AM	AM	AM	AM	AM	AM	PM	PM	PM	PM	PM	PM	PM	PM	PM	PM
Glucose																
A1C1																
Carb Grams																
Fat Grams																
Basal Rate																
Ketones																

NOTES

This is where you tell about the foods that you ate and were not good choices. Tell about your exercise or lack there off. Include details that will reveal the problem areas.

Date: Day:	A M	A M	A M	A M	A M	A M	P M	P M	P M	P M	P M	P M	P M	P M	P M	P M
Glucose																
A1C1																
Carb Grams																
Fat Grams																
Basal Rate																
Ketones																

NOTES

This is where you tell about the foods that you ate and were not good choices. Tell about your exercise or lack there off. Include details that will reveal the problem areas.

Date: Day:	A M	A M	A M	A M	A M	A M	P M	P M	P M	P M	P M	P M	P M	P M	P M	P M
Glucose																
A1C1																
Carb Grams																
Fat Grams																
Basal Rate																
Ketones																

NOTES

This is where you tell about the foods that you ate and were not good choices. Tell about your exercise or lack there off. Include details that will reveal the problem areas.

Date: Day:	A M	A M	A M	A M	A M	A M	P M	P M	P M	P M	P M	P M	P M	P M	P M	P M
Glucose																
A1C1																
Carb Grams																
Fat Grams																
Basal Rate																
Ketones																

NOTES

This is where you tell about the foods that you ate and were not good choices. Tell about your exercise or lack there off. Include details that will reveal the problem areas.

Date: Day:	A M	A M	A M	A M	A M	A M	P M	P M	P M	P M	P M	P M	P M	P M	P M	P M
Glucose																
A1C1																
Carb Grams																
Fat Grams																
Basal Rate																
Ketones																

NOTES
This is where you tell about the foods that you ate and were not good choices. Tell about your exercise or lack there off. Include details that will reveal the problem areas.

Date: Day:	A M	A M	A M	A M	A M	A M	P M	P M	P M	P M	P M	P M	P M	P M	P M	P M
Glucose																
A1C1																
Carb Grams																
Fat Grams																
Basal Rate																
Ketones																

NOTES

This is where you tell about the foods that you ate and were not good choices. Tell about your exercise or lack there off. Include details that will reveal the problem areas.

Date: Day:	A M	A M	A M	A M	A M	A M	P M	P M	P M	P M	P M	P M	P M	P M	P M	P M
Glucose																
A1C1																
Carb Grams																
Fat Grams																
Basal Rate																
Ketones																

NOTES

This is where you tell about the foods that you ate and were not good choices. Tell about your exercise or lack there off. Include details that will reveal the problem areas.

Date: Day:	A M	A M	A M	A M	A M	A M	P M	P M	P M	P M	P M	P M	P M	P M	P M	P M
Glucose																
A1C1																
Carb Grams																
Fat Grams																
Basal Rate																
Ketones																

NOTES

This is where you tell about the foods that you ate and were not good choices. Tell about your exercise or lack there off. Include details that will reveal the problem areas.

Date: Day:	A M	A M	A M	A M	A M	A M	P M	P M	P M	P M	P M	P M	P M	P M	P M	P M
Glucose																
A1C1																
Carb Grams																
Fat Grams																
Basal Rate																
Ketones																

NOTES

This is where you tell about the foods that you ate and were not good choices. Tell about your exercise or lack there off. Include details that will reveal the problem areas.

Date: Day:	A M	A M	A M	A M	A M	A M	P M	P M	P M	P M	P M	P M	P M	P M	P M	P M
Glucose																
A1C1																
Carb Grams																
Fat Grams																
Basal Rate																
Ketones																

NOTES

This is where you tell about the foods that you ate and were not good choices. Tell about your exercise or lack there off. Include details that will reveal the problem areas.

Date: Day:	A M	A M	A M	A M	A M	A M	P M	P M	P M	P M	P M	P M	P M	P M	P M	P M
Glucose																
A1C1																
Carb Grams																
Fat Grams																
Basal Rate																
Ketones																

NOTES

This is where you tell about the foods that you ate and were not good choices. Tell about your exercise or lack there off. Include details that will reveal the problem areas.

Date: Day:	A M	A M	A M	A M	A M	A M	P M	P M	P M	P M	P M	P M	P M	P M	P M	P M
Glucose																
A1C1																
Carb Grams																
Fat Grams																
Basal Rate																
Ketones																

NOTES

This is where you tell about the foods that you ate and were not good choices. Tell about your exercise or lack there off. Include details that will reveal the problem areas.

Date: Day:	A M	A M	A M	A M	A M	A M	P M	P M	P M	P M	P M	P M	P M	P M	P M	P M
Glucose																
A1C1																
Carb Grams																
Fat Grams																
Basal Rate																
Ketones																

NOTES

This is where you tell about the foods that you ate and were not good choices. Tell about your exercise or lack there off. Include details that will reveal the problem areas.

Date: Day:	A M	A M	A M	A M	A M	A M	P M	P M	P M	P M	P M	P M	P M	P M	P M	P M
Glucose																
A1C1																
Carb Grams																
Fat Grams																
Basal Rate																
Ketones																

NOTES

This is where you tell about the foods that you ate and were not good choices. Tell about your exercise or lack there off. Include details that will reveal the problem areas.

Date: Day:	A M	A M	A M	A M	A M	A M	P M	P M	P M	P M	P M	P M	P M	P M	P M	P M
Glucose																
A1C1																
Carb Grams																
Fat Grams																
Basal Rate																
Ketones																

NOTES

This is where you tell about the foods that you ate and were not good choices. Tell about your exercise or lack there off. Include details that will reveal the problem areas.

Date: Day:	A M	A M	A M	A M	A M	A M	P M	P M	P M	P M	P M	P M	P M	P M	P M	P M
Glucose																
A1C1																
Carb Grams																
Fat Grams																
Basal Rate																
Ketones																

NOTES

This is where you tell about the foods that you ate and were not good choices. Tell about your exercise or lack there off. Include details that will reveal the problem areas.

Date: Day:	A M	A M	A M	A M	A M	A M	P M	P M	P M	P M	P M	P M	P M	P M	P M	P M
Glucose																
A1C1																
Carb Grams																
Fat Grams																
Basal Rate																
Ketones																

NOTES

This is where you tell about the foods that you ate and were not good choices. Tell about your exercise or lack there off. Include details that will reveal the problem areas.

Date: Day:	A M	A M	A M	A M	A M	A M	P M	P M	P M	P M	P M	P M	P M	P M	P M	P M
Glucose																
A1C1																
Carb Grams																
Fat Grams																
Basal Rate																
Ketones																

NOTES
This is where you tell about the foods that you ate and were not good choices. Tell about your exercise or lack there off. Include details that will reveal the problem areas.

Date: Day:	A M	A M	A M	A M	A M	A M	P M	P M	P M	P M	P M	P M	P M	P M	P M	P M
Glucose																
A1C1																
Carb Grams																
Fat Grams																
Basal Rate																
Ketones																

NOTES

This is where you tell about the foods that you ate and were not good choices. Tell about your exercise or lack there off. Include details that will reveal the problem areas.

Date: Day:	A M	A M	A M	A M	A M	A M	P M	P M	P M	P M	P M	P M	P M	P M	P M	P M
Glucose																
A1C1																
Carb Grams																
Fat Grams																
Basal Rate																
Ketones																

NOTES

This is where you tell about the foods that you ate and were not good choices. Tell about your exercise or lack there off. Include details that will reveal the problem areas.

Date: Day:	A M	A M	A M	A M	A M	A M	P M	P M	P M	P M	P M	P M	P M	P M	P M	P M
Glucose																
A1C1																
Carb Grams																
Fat Grams																
Basal Rate																
Ketones																

NOTES

This is where you tell about the foods that you ate and were not good choices. Tell about your exercise or lack there off. Include details that will reveal the problem areas.

Date: Day:	A M	A M	A M	A M	A M	A M	P M	P M	P M	P M	P M	P M	P M	P M	P M	P M
Glucose																
A1C1																
Carb Grams																
Fat Grams																
Basal Rate																
Ketones																

NOTES

This is where you tell about the foods that you ate and were not good choices. Tell about your exercise or lack there off. Include details that will reveal the problem areas.

Date: Day:	A M	A M	A M	A M	A M	A M	P M	P M	P M	P M	P M	P M	P M	P M	P M	P M
Glucose																
A1C1																
Carb Grams																
Fat Grams																
Basal Rate																
Ketones																

NOTES
This is where you tell about the foods that you ate and
were not good choices. Tell about your exercise or lack
there off. Include details that will reveal the problem areas.

Date: Day:	A M	A M	A M	A M	A M	A M	P M	P M	P M	P M	P M	P M	P M	P M	P M	P M
Glucose																
A1C1																
Carb Grams																
Fat Grams																
Basal Rate																
Ketones																

NOTES
This is where you tell about the foods that you ate and
were not good choices. Tell about your exercise or lack
there off. Include details that will reveal the problem areas.

Date: Day:	A M	A M	A M	A M	A M	A M	P M	P M	P M	P M	P M	P M	P M	P M	P M	P M
Glucose																
A1C1																
Carb Grams																
Fat Grams																
Basal Rate																
Ketones																

NOTES

This is where you tell about the foods that you ate and were not good choices. Tell about your exercise or lack there off. Include details that will reveal the problem areas.

Date: Day:	A M	A M	A M	A M	A M	A M	P M	P M	P M	P M	P M	P M	P M	P M	P M	P M
Glucose																
A1C1																
Carb Grams																
Fat Grams																
Basal Rate																
Ketones																

NOTES

This is where you tell about the foods that you ate and were not good choices. Tell about your exercise or lack there off. Include details that will reveal the problem areas.

Date: Day:	A M	A M	A M	A M	A M	A M	P M	P M	P M	P M	P M	P M	P M	P M	P M	P M
Glucose																
A1C1																
Carb Grams																
Fat Grams																
Basal Rate																
Ketones																

NOTES

This is where you tell about the foods that you ate and were not good choices. Tell about your exercise or lack there off. Include details that will reveal the problem areas.

Date: Day:	A M	A M	A M	A M	A M	A M	P M	P M	P M	P M	P M	P M	P M	P M	P M	P M
Glucose																
A1C1																
Carb Grams																
Fat Grams																
Basal Rate																
Ketones																

NOTES

This is where you tell about the foods that you ate and were not good choices. Tell about your exercise or lack there off. Include details that will reveal the problem areas.

Date: Day:	A M	A M	A M	A M	A M	A M	P M	P M	P M	P M	P M	P M	P M	P M	P M	P M
Glucose																
A1C1																
Carb Grams																
Fat Grams																
Basal Rate																
Ketones																

MONTH FIVE

Congratulation on your perseverance and keep it up. The prize is ahead and it is better health and a longer life.

NOTES

This is where you tell about the foods that you ate and were not good choices. Tell about your exercise or lack there off. Include details that will reveal the problem areas.

Date: Day:	A M	A M	A M	A M	A M	A M	P M	P M	P M	P M	P M	P M	P M	P M	P M	P M
Glucose																
A1C1																
Carb Grams																
Fat Grams																
Basal Rate																
Ketones																

NOTES

This is where you tell about the foods that you ate and were not good choices. Tell about your exercise or lack there off. Include details that will reveal the problem areas.

Date: Day:	A M	A M	A M	A M	A M	A M	P M	P M	P M	P M	P M	P M	P M	P M	P M	P M
Glucose																
A1C1																
Carb Grams																
Fat Grams																
Basal Rate																
Ketones																

NOTES

This is where you tell about the foods that you ate and were not good choices. Tell about your exercise or lack there off. Include details that will reveal the problem areas.

Date: Day:	A M	A M	A M	A M	A M	A M	P M	P M	P M	P M	P M	P M	P M	P M	P M	P M
Glucose																
A1C1																
Carb Grams																
Fat Grams																
Basal Rate																
Ketones																

NOTES

This is where you tell about the foods that you ate and were not good choices. Tell about your exercise or lack there off. Include details that will reveal the problem areas.

Date: Day:	A M	A M	A M	A M	A M	A M	P M	P M	P M	P M	P M	P M	P M	P M	P M	P M
Glucose																
A1C1																
Carb Grams																
Fat Grams																
Basal Rate																
Ketones																

NOTES

This is where you tell about the foods that you ate and were not good choices. Tell about your exercise or lack there off. Include details that will reveal the problem areas.

Date: Day:	A M	A M	A M	A M	A M	A M	P M	P M	P M	P M	P M	P M	P M	P M	P M	P M
Glucose																
A1C1																
Carb Grams																
Fat Grams																
Basal Rate																
Ketones																

NOTES

This is where you tell about the foods that you ate and were not good choices. Tell about your exercise or lack there off. Include details that will reveal the problem areas.

Date: Day:	A M	A M	A M	A M	A M	A M	P M	P M	P M	P M	P M	P M	P M	P M	P M	P M
Glucose																
A1C1																
Carb Grams																
Fat Grams																
Basal Rate																
Ketones																

NOTES
This is where you tell about the foods that you ate and were not good choices. Tell about your exercise or lack there off. Include details that will reveal the problem areas.

Date: Day:	A M	A M	A M	A M	A M	A M	P M	P M	P M	P M	P M	P M	P M	P M	P M	P M
Glucose																
A1C1																
Carb Grams																
Fat Grams																
Basal Rate																
Ketones																

NOTES

This is where you tell about the foods that you ate and were not good choices. Tell about your exercise or lack there off. Include details that will reveal the problem areas.

Date: Day:	A M	A M	A M	A M	A M	A M	P M	P M	P M	P M	P M	P M	P M	P M	P M	P M
Glucose																
A1C1																
Carb Grams																
Fat Grams																
Basal Rate																
Ketones																

NOTES

This is where you tell about the foods that you ate and were not good choices. Tell about your exercise or lack there off. Include details that will reveal the problem areas.

Date: Day:	A M	A M	A M	A M	A M	A M	P M	P M	P M	P M	P M	P M	P M	P M	P M	P M
Glucose																
A1C1																
Carb Grams																
Fat Grams																
Basal Rate																
Ketones																

NOTES

This is where you tell about the foods that you ate and were not good choices. Tell about your exercise or lack there off. Include details that will reveal the problem areas.

Date: Day:	A M	A M	A M	A M	A M	A M	P M	P M	P M	P M	P M	P M	P M	P M	P M	P M
Glucose																
A1C1																
Carb Grams																
Fat Grams																
Basal Rate																
Ketones																

NOTES

This is where you tell about the foods that you ate and were not good choices. Tell about your exercise or lack there off. Include details that will reveal the problem areas.

Date: Day:	A M	A M	A M	A M	A M	A M	P M	P M	P M	P M	P M	P M	P M	P M	P M	P M
Glucose																
A1C1																
Carb Grams																
Fat Grams																
Basal Rate																
Ketones																

NOTES

This is where you tell about the foods that you ate and were not good choices. Tell about your exercise or lack there off. Include details that will reveal the problem areas.

Date: Day:	A M	A M	A M	A M	A M	A M	P M	P M	P M	P M	P M	P M	P M	P M	P M	P M
Glucose																
A1C1																
Carb Grams																
Fat Grams																
Basal Rate																
Ketones																

NOTES

This is where you tell about the foods that you ate and were not good choices. Tell about your exercise or lack there off. Include details that will reveal the problem areas.

Date: Day:	A M	A M	A M	A M	A M	A M	P M	P M	P M	P M	P M	P M	P M	P M	P M	P M
Glucose																
A1C1																
Carb Grams																
Fat Grams																
Basal Rate																
Ketones																

NOTES

This is where you tell about the foods that you ate and were not good choices. Tell about your exercise or lack there off. Include details that will reveal the problem areas.

Date: Day:	A M	A M	A M	A M	A M	A M	P M	P M	P M	P M	P M	P M	P M	P M	P M	P M
Glucose																
A1C1																
Carb Grams																
Fat Grams																
Basal Rate																
Ketones																

NOTES
This is where you tell about the foods that you ate and were not good choices. Tell about your exercise or lack there off. Include details that will reveal the problem areas.

Date: Day:	A M	A M	A M	A M	A M	A M	P M	P M	P M	P M	P M	P M	P M	P M	P M	P M
Glucose																
A1C1																
Carb Grams																
Fat Grams																
Basal Rate																
Ketones																

NOTES

This is where you tell about the foods that you ate and were not good choices. Tell about your exercise or lack there off. Include details that will reveal the problem areas.

Date: Day:	A M	A M	A M	A M	A M	A M	P M	P M	P M	P M	P M	P M	P M	P M	P M	P M
Glucose																
A1C1																
Carb Grams																
Fat Grams																
Basal Rate																
Ketones																

NOTES
This is where you tell about the foods that you ate and were not good choices. Tell about your exercise or lack there off. Include details that will reveal the problem areas.

Date: Day:	A M	A M	A M	A M	A M	A M	P M	P M	P M	P M	P M	P M	P M	P M	P M	P M
Glucose																
A1C1																
Carb Grams																
Fat Grams																
Basal Rate																
Ketones																

NOTES

This is where you tell about the foods that you ate and were not good choices. Tell about your exercise or lack there off. Include details that will reveal the problem areas.

Date: Day:	A M	A M	A M	A M	A M	A M	P M	P M	P M	P M	P M	P M	P M	P M	P M	P M
Glucose																
A1C1																
Carb Grams																
Fat Grams																
Basal Rate																
Ketones																

NOTES
This is where you tell about the foods that you ate and were not good choices. Tell about your exercise or lack there off. Include details that will reveal the problem areas.

Date: Day:	A M	A M	A M	A M	A M	A M	P M	P M	P M	P M	P M	P M	P M	P M	P M	P M
Glucose																
A1C1																
Carb Grams																
Fat Grams																
Basal Rate																
Ketones																

NOTES

This is where you tell about the foods that you ate and were not good choices. Tell about your exercise or lack there off. Include details that will reveal the problem areas.

Date: Day:	A M	A M	A M	A M	A M	A M	P M	P M	P M	P M	P M	P M	P M	P M	P M	P M
Glucose																
A1C1																
Carb Grams																
Fat Grams																
Basal Rate																
Ketones																

NOTES
This is where you tell about the foods that you ate and were not good choices. Tell about your exercise or lack there off. Include details that will reveal the problem areas.

Date: Day:	A M	A M	A M	A M	A M	A M	P M	P M	P M	P M	P M	P M	P M	P M	P M	P M
Glucose																
A1C1																
Carb Grams																
Fat Grams																
Basal Rate																
Ketones																

NOTES

This is where you tell about the foods that you ate and were not good choices. Tell about your exercise or lack there off. Include details that will reveal the problem areas.

Date: Day:	A M	A M	A M	A M	A M	A M	P M	P M	P M	P M	P M	P M	P M	P M	P M	P M
Glucose																
A1C1																
Carb Grams																
Fat Grams																
Basal Rate																
Ketones																

NOTES

This is where you tell about the foods that you ate and were not good choices. Tell about your exercise or lack there off. Include details that will reveal the problem areas.

Date: Day:	A M	A M	A M	A M	A M	A M	P M	P M	P M	P M	P M	P M	P M	P M	P M	P M
Glucose																
A1C1																
Carb Grams																
Fat Grams																
Basal Rate																
Ketones																

NOTES

This is where you tell about the foods that you ate and were not good choices. Tell about your exercise or lack there off. Include details that will reveal the problem areas.

Date: Day:	A M	A M	A M	A M	A M	A M	P M	P M	P M	P M	P M	P M	P M	P M	P M	P M
Glucose																
A1C1																
Carb Grams																
Fat Grams																
Basal Rate																
Ketones																

NOTES

This is where you tell about the foods that you ate and were not good choices. Tell about your exercise or lack there off. Include details that will reveal the problem areas.

Date: Day:	A M	A M	A M	A M	A M	A M	P M	P M	P M	P M	P M	P M	P M	P M	P M	P M
Glucose																
A1C1																
Carb Grams																
Fat Grams																
Basal Rate																
Ketones																

NOTES

This is where you tell about the foods that you ate and were not good choices. Tell about your exercise or lack there off. Include details that will reveal the problem areas.

Date: Day:	A M	A M	A M	A M	A M	A M	P M	P M	P M	P M	P M	P M	P M	P M	P M	P M
Glucose																
A1C1																
Carb Grams																
Fat Grams																
Basal Rate																
Ketones																

NOTES

This is where you tell about the foods that you ate and were not good choices. Tell about your exercise or lack there off. Include details that will reveal the problem areas.

Date: Day:	A M	A M	A M	A M	A M	A M	P M	P M	P M	P M	P M	P M	P M	P M	P M	P M
Glucose																
A1C1																
Carb Grams																
Fat Grams																
Basal Rate																
Ketones																

NOTES

This is where you tell about the foods that you ate and were not good choices. Tell about your exercise or lack there off. Include details that will reveal the problem areas.

Date: Day:	A M	A M	A M	A M	A M	A M	P M	P M	P M	P M	P M	P M	P M	P M	P M	P M
Glucose																
A1C1																
Carb Grams																
Fat Grams																
Basal Rate																
Ketones																

NOTES

This is where you tell about the foods that you ate and were not good choices. Tell about your exercise or lack there off. Include details that will reveal the problem areas.

Date: Day:	A M	A M	A M	A M	A M	A M	P M	P M	P M	P M	P M	P M	P M	P M	P M	P M
Glucose																
A1C1																
Carb Grams																
Fat Grams																
Basal Rate																
Ketones																

NOTES

This is where you tell about the foods that you ate and were not good choices. Tell about your exercise or lack there off. Include details that will reveal the problem areas.

Date: Day:	A M	A M	A M	A M	A M	A M	P M	P M	P M	P M	P M	P M	P M	P M	P M	P M
Glucose																
A1C1																
Carb Grams																
Fat Grams																
Basal Rate																
Ketones																

NOTES

This is where you tell about the foods that you ate and were not good choices. Tell about your exercise or lack there off. Include details that will reveal the problem areas.

Date: Day:	A M	A M	A M	A M	A M	A M	P M	P M	P M	P M	P M	P M	P M	P M	P M	P M
Glucose																
A1C1																
Carb Grams																
Fat Grams																
Basal Rate																
Ketones																

MONTH SIX

Congratulations you have completed your first month. How did you do with your data? Keep up the great work and be consistent and there will be results in improved glucose and better health.

NOTES

This is where you tell about the foods that you ate and were not good choices. Tell about your exercise or lack there off. Include details that will reveal the problem areas.

Date: Day:	A M	A M	A M	A M	A M	A M	P M	P M	P M	P M	P M	P M	P M	P M	P M	P M
Glucose																
A1C1																
Carb Grams																
Fat Grams																
Basal Rate																
Ketones																

NOTES

This is where you tell about the foods that you ate and were not good choices. Tell about your exercise or lack there off. Include details that will reveal the problem areas.

Date: Day:	A M	A M	A M	A M	A M	A M	P M	P M	P M	P M	P M	P M	P M	P M	P M	P M
Glucose																
A1C1																
Carb Grams																
Fat Grams																
Basal Rate																
Ketones																

NOTES

This is where you tell about the foods that you ate and were not good choices. Tell about your exercise or lack there off. Include details that will reveal the problem areas.

Date: Day:	A M	A M	A M	A M	A M	A M	P M	P M	P M	P M	P M	P M	P M	P M	P M	P M
Glucose																
A1C1																
Carb Grams																
Fat Grams																
Basal Rate																
Ketones																

NOTES

This is where you tell about the foods that you ate and were not good choices. Tell about your exercise or lack there off. Include details that will reveal the problem areas.

Date: Day:	A M	A M	A M	A M	A M	A M	P M	P M	P M	P M	P M	P M	P M	P M	P M	P M
Glucose																
A1C1																
Carb Grams																
Fat Grams																
Basal Rate																
Ketones																

NOTES
This is where you tell about the foods that you ate and were not good choices. Tell about your exercise or lack there off. Include details that will reveal the problem areas.

Date: Day:	A M	A M	A M	A M	A M	A M	P M	P M	P M	P M	P M	P M	P M	P M	P M	P M
Glucose																
A1C1																
Carb Grams																
Fat Grams																
Basal Rate																
Ketones																

NOTES

This is where you tell about the foods that you ate and were not good choices. Tell about your exercise or lack there off. Include details that will reveal the problem areas.

Date: Day:	A M	A M	A M	A M	A M	A M	P M	P M	P M	P M	P M	P M	P M	P M	P M	P M
Glucose																
A1C1																
Carb Grams																
Fat Grams																
Basal Rate																
Ketones																

NOTES

This is where you tell about the foods that you ate and were not good choices. Tell about your exercise or lack there off. Include details that will reveal the problem areas.

Date: Day:	A M	A M	A M	A M	A M	A M	P M	P M	P M	P M	P M	P M	P M	P M	P M	P M
Glucose																
A1C1																
Carb Grams																
Fat Grams																
Basal Rate																
Ketones																

NOTES
This is where you tell about the foods that you ate and were not good choices. Tell about your exercise or lack there off. Include details that will reveal the problem areas.

Date: Day:	A M	A M	A M	A M	A M	A M	P M	P M	P M	P M	P M	P M	P M	P M	P M	P M
Glucose																
A1C1																
Carb Grams																
Fat Grams																
Basal Rate																
Ketones																

NOTES
This is where you tell about the foods that you ate and were not good choices. Tell about your exercise or lack there off. Include details that will reveal the problem areas.

Date: Day:	A M	A M	A M	A M	A M	A M	P M	P M	P M	P M	P M	P M	P M	P M	P M	P M
Glucose																
A1C1																
Carb Grams																
Fat Grams																
Basal Rate																
Ketones																

NOTES
This is where you tell about the foods that you ate and were not good choices. Tell about your exercise or lack there off. Include details that will reveal the problem areas.

Date: Day:	A M	A M	A M	A M	A M	A M	P M	P M	P M	P M	P M	P M	P M	P M	P M	P M
Glucose																
A1C1																
Carb Grams																
Fat Grams																
Basal Rate																
Ketones																

NOTES

This is where you tell about the foods that you ate and were not good choices. Tell about your exercise or lack there off. Include details that will reveal the problem areas.

Date: Day:	A M	A M	A M	A M	A M	A M	P M	P M	P M	P M	P M	P M	P M	P M	P M	P M
Glucose																
A1C1																
Carb Grams																
Fat Grams																
Basal Rate																
Ketones																

NOTES
This is where you tell about the foods that you ate and were not good choices. Tell about your exercise or lack there off. Include details that will reveal the problem areas.

Date: Day:	A M	A M	A M	A M	A M	A M	P M	P M	P M	P M	P M	P M	P M	P M	P M	P M
Glucose																
A1C1																
Carb Grams																
Fat Grams																
Basal Rate																
Ketones																

NOTES

This is where you tell about the foods that you ate and were not good choices. Tell about your exercise or lack there off. Include details that will reveal the problem areas.

Date: Day:	A M	A M	A M	A M	A M	A M	P M	P M	P M	P M	P M	P M	P M	P M	P M	P M
Glucose																
A1C1																
Carb Grams																
Fat Grams																
Basal Rate																
Ketones																

NOTES

This is where you tell about the foods that you ate and were not good choices. Tell about your exercise or lack there off. Include details that will reveal the problem areas.

Date: Day:	A M	A M	A M	A M	A M	A M	P M	P M	P M	P M	P M	P M	P M	P M	P M	P M
Glucose																
A1C1																
Carb Grams																
Fat Grams																
Basal Rate																
Ketones																

NOTES
This is where you tell about the foods that you ate and were not good choices. Tell about your exercise or lack there off. Include details that will reveal the problem areas.

Date: Day:	A M	A M	A M	A M	A M	A M	P M	P M	P M	P M	P M	P M	P M	P M	P M	P M
Glucose																
A1C1																
Carb Grams																
Fat Grams																
Basal Rate																
Ketones																

NOTES
This is where you tell about the foods that you ate and were not good choices. Tell about your exercise or lack there off. Include details that will reveal the problem areas.

Date: Day:	A M	A M	A M	A M	A M	A M	P M	P M	P M	P M	P M	P M	P M	P M	P M	P M
Glucose																
A1C1																
Carb Grams																
Fat Grams																
Basal Rate																
Ketones																

NOTES

This is where you tell about the foods that you ate and were not good choices. Tell about your exercise or lack there off. Include details that will reveal the problem areas.

Date: Day:	A M	A M	A M	A M	A M	A M	P M	P M	P M	P M	P M	P M	P M	P M	P M	P M
Glucose																
A1C1																
Carb Grams																
Fat Grams																
Basal Rate																
Ketones																

NOTES

This is where you tell about the foods that you ate and were not good choices. Tell about your exercise or lack there off. Include details that will reveal the problem areas.

Date: Day:	A M	A M	A M	A M	A M	A M	P M	P M	P M	P M	P M	P M	P M	P M	P M	P M
Glucose																
A1C1																
Carb Grams																
Fat Grams																
Basal Rate																
Ketones																

NOTES

This is where you tell about the foods that you ate and were not good choices. Tell about your exercise or lack there off. Include details that will reveal the problem areas.

Date: Day:	A M	A M	A M	A M	A M	A M	P M	P M	P M	P M	P M	P M	P M	P M	P M	P M
Glucose																
A1C1																
Carb Grams																
Fat Grams																
Basal Rate																
Ketones																

NOTES

This is where you tell about the foods that you ate and were not good choices. Tell about your exercise or lack there off. Include details that will reveal the problem areas.

Date: Day:	A M	A M	A M	A M	A M	A M	P M	P M	P M	P M	P M	P M	P M	P M	P M	P M
Glucose																
A1C1																
Carb Grams																
Fat Grams																
Basal Rate																
Ketones																

NOTES

This is where you tell about the foods that you ate and were not good choices. Tell about your exercise or lack there off. Include details that will reveal the problem areas.

Date: Day:	A M	A M	A M	A M	A M	A M	P M	P M	P M	P M	P M	P M	P M	P M	P M	P M
Glucose																
A1C1																
Carb Grams																
Fat Grams																
Basal Rate																
Ketones																

NOTES

This is where you tell about the foods that you ate and were not good choices. Tell about your exercise or lack there off. Include details that will reveal the problem areas.

Date: Day:	A M	A M	A M	A M	A M	A M	P M	P M	P M	P M	P M	P M	P M	P M	P M	P M
Glucose																
A1C1																
Carb Grams																
Fat Grams																
Basal Rate																
Ketones																

NOTES

This is where you tell about the foods that you ate and were not good choices. Tell about your exercise or lack there off. Include details that will reveal the problem areas.

Date: Day:	A M	A M	A M	A M	A M	A M	P M	P M	P M	P M	P M	P M	P M	P M	P M	P M
Glucose																
A1C1																
Carb Grams																
Fat Grams																
Basal Rate																
Ketones																

NOTES

This is where you tell about the foods that you ate and were not good choices. Tell about your exercise or lack there off. Include details that will reveal the problem areas.

Date: Day:	AM	AM	AM	AM	AM	AM	PM	PM	PM	PM	PM	PM	PM	PM	PM	PM
Glucose																
A1C1																
Carb Grams																
Fat Grams																
Basal Rate																
Ketones																

NOTES

This is where you tell about the foods that you ate and were not good choices. Tell about your exercise or lack there off. Include details that will reveal the problem areas.

Date: Day:	A M	A M	A M	A M	A M	A M	P M	P M	P M	P M	P M	P M	P M	P M	P M	P M
Glucose																
A1C1																
Carb Grams																
Fat Grams																
Basal Rate																
Ketones																

NOTES

This is where you tell about the foods that you ate and were not good choices. Tell about your exercise or lack there off. Include details that will reveal the problem areas.

Date: Day:	A M	A M	A M	A M	A M	A M	P M	P M	P M	P M	P M	P M	P M	P M	P M	P M
Glucose																
A1C1																
Carb Grams																
Fat Grams																
Basal Rate																
Ketones																

NOTES

This is where you tell about the foods that you ate and were not good choices. Tell about your exercise or lack there off. Include details that will reveal the problem areas.

Date: Day:	A M	A M	A M	A M	A M	A M	P M	P M	P M	P M	P M	P M	P M	P M	P M	P M
Glucose																
A1C1																
Carb Grams																
Fat Grams																
Basal Rate																
Ketones																

NOTES

This is where you tell about the foods that you ate and were not good choices. Tell about your exercise or lack there off. Include details that will reveal the problem areas.

Date: Day:	A M	A M	A M	A M	A M	A M	P M	P M	P M	P M	P M	P M	P M	P M	P M	P M
Glucose																
A1C1																
Carb Grams																
Fat Grams																
Basal Rate																
Ketones																

NOTES
This is where you tell about the foods that you ate and were not good choices. Tell about your exercise or lack there off. Include details that will reveal the problem areas.

Date: Day:	A M	A M	A M	A M	A M	A M	P M	P M	P M	P M	P M	P M	P M	P M	P M	P M
Glucose																
A1C1																
Carb Grams																
Fat Grams																
Basal Rate																
Ketones																

NOTES

This is where you tell about the foods that you ate and were not good choices. Tell about your exercise or lack there off. Include details that will reveal the problem areas.

Date: Day:	A M	A M	A M	A M	A M	A M	P M	P M	P M	P M	P M	P M	P M	P M	P M	P M
Glucose																
A1C1																
Carb Grams																
Fat Grams																
Basal Rate																
Ketones																

NOTES

This is where you tell about the foods that you ate and were not good choices. Tell about your exercise or lack there off. Include details that will reveal the problem areas.

Date: Day:	A M	A M	A M	A M	A M	A M	P M	P M	P M	P M	P M	P M	P M	P M	P M	P M
Glucose																
A1C1																
Carb Grams																
Fat Grams																
Basal Rate																
Ketones																

7 CONCLUSION

So you have two 90 day time frames to document your daily data and can look for any patterns that will indicate where the areas are that will allow you to tweak your diet and lifestyle to improve your Diabetic health.

Jot down your goals for the next 90 days and let us begin again, looking for even more results!

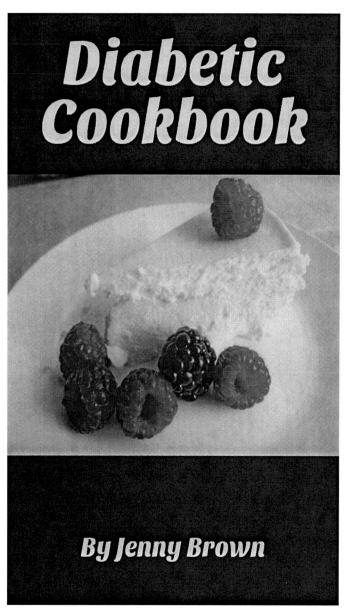

Diabetic Cookbook

By Jenny Brown

Comments from your physician

Write down the recommendations that your doctors makes at each and every visit.

Make notes on questions that you may have before your next visit with your doctor.

CPSIA information can be obtained at www.ICGtesting.com
Printed in the USA
LVOW13s2344160714

394642LV00030B/1077/P